I WANT TO
VAPE!

DONALD BLAKELY

I WANT TO VAPE!

ELECTRONIC CIGARETTE AND VAPING BEGINNERS GUIDE

Miller Creative
Publishing

I Want to Vape!

First Edition, January2015

Easy Vaping Guides
www.evguides.co.uk

Miller Creative Publishing
www.millercp.co.uk

Paperback ISBN: 978-1505871791

CONTENTS

Getting Started

The Electronic Cigarette

Cartomisers, Clearomisers & RBAs

Accessories

E-liquid

And Finally...

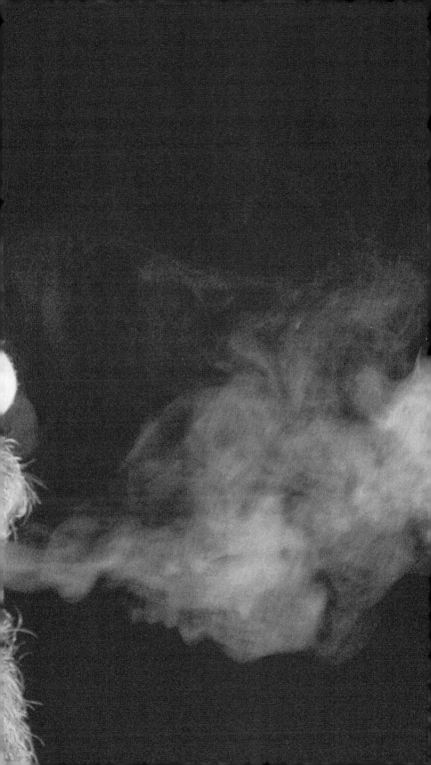

GETTING STARTED

1 Introduction

We all know that smoking is bad for your body. It destroys your airways, hardening and blackening the soft tissues in your lungs. It destroys your skin and makes you look old faster; causing wrinkles and toughening your skin.

It can cause **cancer**, erectile dysfunction, glaucoma, cataracts, infertility as well as a host of other health issues.

Do you want to be smoking tobacco cigarettes?

There's no denying that electronic cigarettes have had a major impact on the lives of many smokers; myself included! And with electronic cigarettes featuring more and more in the news and vaping becoming more common around the world it's only natural that more and more people are making the switch to electronic cigarettes and a healthier life.

Maybe you want to make your purchases before any new regulations kick in (actually limiting your choices), or maybe you want to quit smoking, help someone else to quit or you just want a better understanding of electronic cigarettes.

There's a mountain of equipment, e-liquid and accessories to choose from and so much information to sift through.

But where do you start?

You need answers and you don't have time to search the Internet or interview experienced vapers. You may not even know what information to search for.

Well there's no need to search around! You've bought this comprehensive guide; the first in a series of books written in order to help you fully understand vaping.

By the end you'll be able to identify the various types of devices available, make informed decisions on your purchases and understand any health or safety issues.

Not every topic covered in this book could have its own heading in the contents list; so you'll discover some hidden nuggets of information that no one thinks to mention when you start vaping; so you'll know what to expect.

Don't worry! I'm not going to bombard you with technical jargon!

There are many acronyms in the vaping world, but by the end of this book (and this series) you'll be familiar with all of these terms.

So why did I write this book?

Vaping saved my life, but I found that the journey to finding all of the relevant information was long and at times costly, due to mistakes or misinformation. I want to share my knowledge with you (just as I have with my family and friends) and make your vaping experience **great from the start**.

In the past I tried to quit smoking by using various NRT products, chewing gum and willpower. I can't resist chocolate let alone a cigarette, so willpower was a total fail. All my attempts to quit smoking were unsuccessful until I discovered electronic cigarettes.

I have never looked back!

My health has improved, my clothes and home don't smell like ashtrays anymore and I have more money (I'll admit I spend a lot of that saving on more vaping equipment). My sense of smell has returned and as for my taste buds... well! They're jumping for joy!

If you're looking to make the change to electronic cigarettes, all I can say is...

...Welcome to the wonderful world of vaping!

2 History of Electronic Cigarettes

Electronic cigarettes have been around for a very long time but it's only recently that they have become popular due to the growing number of people using them to stop smoking or to continue with nicotine but cut out the harmful chemicals contained within tobacco cigarettes.

So how did it all begin?

Before we rush into the main inventors there is an inventor called Joseph Robinson that is often overlooked when we talk about the history of electronic cigarettes.

Maybe it's because his idea was not designed to be a 'tobacco alternative', but an 'Electric Vaporiser' designed for holding medicinal compounds.

Back in 1930, Joseph's patent was approved for a device that could be 'freely handled without possibility of being burned', that would electrically heat medicinal compounds that would produce vapour for inhalation.

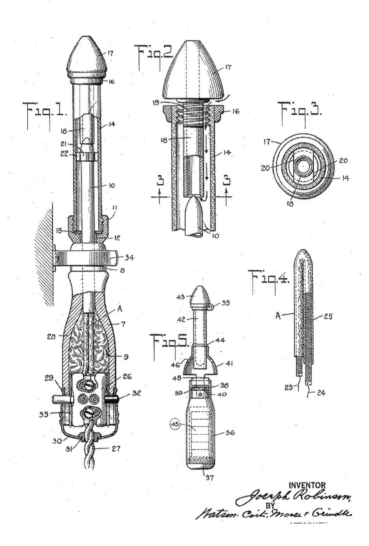

INVENTOR

Joseph Robinson,

BY

Watson, Coit, Morse & Grindle

As you can see there are so many similarities to electronic cigarettes in his invention; you can see why he needed to be mentioned; as this surely would have influenced earlier designs. It was an inventor named Herbert Gilbert who first envisaged the idea of a 'tobacco alternative' device in 1963.

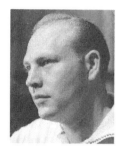

His patent (filed in Pennsylvania) for a 'Smokeless Non Tobacco Cigarette' was approved in 1965. Nearly fifty years ago! Now although several companies approached him to develop his idea, nothing emerged or progressed.

Why?

Well after several discussions, the companies decided to wait for the patent to expire; so that they could develop their own products and 'cut out' Herbert.

I know... business right!

Now even though Herbert had the idea initially he is not the person internationally recognised for developing the actual modern electronic cigarettes that we see today.

Between 1965 and 2000, there are a lot more patents filed in relation to electronic cigarette devices. There are too many for me to go through here; and not really relevant as none of them were developed.

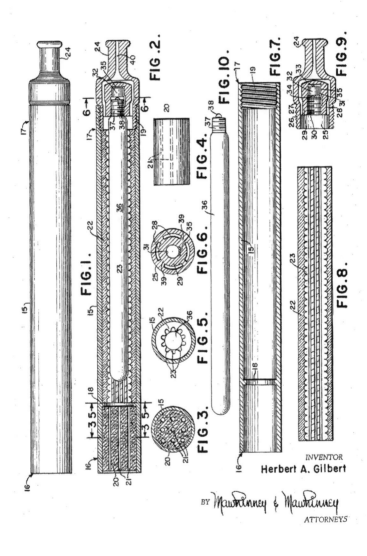

FIG.2.
FIG.7.
FIG.9.
FIG.10.
FIG.4.
FIG.1.
FIG.6.
FIG.5.
FIG.3.
FIG.8.

INVENTOR
Herbert A. Gilbert

BY Mawhinney & Mawhinney
ATTORNEYS

So who got the ball rolling?

It was a chemist named Hon Lik who designed a device in the year 2000. His development of the device was fuelled by his father developing lung cancer from smoking. Hon was also a smoker, smoking sixty a day.

Now Hon states that his idea for an electronic cigarette came to him in a dream. In his dream he states that he was coughing and wheezing and he imagined himself drowning. The water around him lifted, turning into a cloud of vapour. This gave him the inspiration for the device; which he scribbled down.

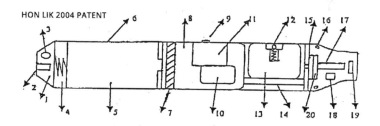

Hon's device was the basis of what we see today; a mouthpiece, battery and atomiser. In more detail it was a small plastic tank with a mouthpiece which held a nicotine and 'propylene glycol' mixture. A piezoelectric ultrasonic element was used to vaporise the mixture by creating a pressurised jet of the liquid.

Now Hon's involvement did not stop there; he refined the device. And after he filed for a patent in early 2004 (through his company 'Golden Dragon Holdings'), the first devices that we recognise today was introduced to the Chinese market later that year.

He later went on to change the name of the company to 'Ruyan' which means 'resembling smoking'. Ruyan started exporting the devices in 2005 and the company received their first international patent in 2007.

Today electronic cigarettes have caused somewhat of a stir worldwide. Due to its popularity and its similarity to smoking, bans on 'public vaping' have been exercised in many countries.

In places where bans have been imposed vapers can only vape in areas designated to smokers. And many workplaces are now editing their work policies to exclude vaping in the workplace.

The exact future direction of electronic cigarettes at this present moment is not looking too good. With calls for electronic cigarettes and e-liquid to be heavily regulated on an international level.

Some countries have implemented a complete ban on all electronic cigarettes and e-liquid. But we won't go into the politics of it all in this book.

3 Vaping Guide

So what exactly is vaping?

Let's put this simply... if you exhale smoke, you are smoking, if you exhale vapour you are vaping!

Vaping is when you use an electronic cigarette or personal vaporiser (same thing) to deliver nicotine. If you vape then you are referred to as a vaper.

If you are (or were) a smoker, do you remember the first puff you took of a cigarette? Do you remember coughing or even gagging? Well that was your body adjusting to smoking for the first time. After a while you got use to smoking.

Well the same thing normally happens when you start vaping. It's something new to your body, which has become accustomed to tobacco smoke.

The vapour you inhale is not dry like tobacco smoke, it has a slightly wet feeling and your body will think "What is this... get it out?" and cause you to cough or gag; which is all very natural and does not last for long.

Actually the first recorded reference to vaping and vapers was by a Dr Norman L Jacobson back in 1981, over 30 years ago.

Vaping is not smoking!

When you are vaping you are inhaling the vapour produced from an electronic cigarette by the heating of a small amount of liquid; as opposed to inhaling smoke from a tobacco cigarette created by combustion (burning).

So vaping is not smoking! It is the inhalation of vapour. The taste is different; the amount of vapour produced is far cleaner, superior and thicker to that of smoking.

And the smell, well... most of the time there is no smell or if there is the worst you will get is air filled with a banana scent, coffee, vanilla or whatever flavour you are vaping.

In fact the only real similarities to smoking are that you inhale, exhale and take in nicotine.

If you were (or are) a smoker, you've probably spent years abusing your senses, so much to the point that you are used to the chemical taste of cigarettes.

When you stop smoking your senses start to heal. You start to taste your food again and your sense of smell returns.

In fact you might be tempted to think you have gained super powers when you can smell a cigarette being smoked far off into the distance, out of sight.

The smell of a cigarette (that little stick that you once craved and loved) might even start to make you feel slightly sick.

Say goodbye to 'that' smell

A while after I had quit smoking I was travelling on a bus and a woman got on and sat next to me. She absolutely 'reeked' of cigarette smoke. All I could think was "did I really use to smell like that?"

I believe it was so obvious to her that my senses had been 'invaded' because she reached into her bag, popped a few mints into her mouth and crossed her arms to close her jacket.

I felt bad for her and slightly ashamed, as I knew the same 'polite' look that I (and others) had given her was the same that I had received for many years.

But let's face it... cigarettes smell (and taste) bad! And there's no hiding!

Is Vaping Safe?

Anything that contains nicotine cannot be stated as 100% safe. However, evidence strongly suggests that vaping is far safer than smoking tobacco cigarettes.

Experts have shown that switching from smoking to vaping reduces health risks to less than 1% of smoking tobacco cigarettes (nearly the same as non-smokers). So we can safely say that...

...Vaping is 99% safer than smoking.

Can vaping cause cancer?

Ok... The truth! The FDA did find 'trace amounts' of tobacco specific nitrosamines (carcinogens) in electronic cigarettes, which are known to cause cancer with high exposure, but the levels found were 'extremely' low.

The FDA did not release any figures for the levels that they found... hmm! But if we look at the scientific definition of 'trace amounts' it means 'amounts that are detectable, but too small to accurately measure'.

Let's not panic though!

If you're now standing over a bin, about to throw away your electronic cigarette... DON'T!

Worldwide food organisations actually allow certain levels of nitrosamines in consumable products. Do a quick Google search. You'll find it in toothpaste, meat, beer (aww!), cosmetics, chocolate (noooooo!) and more.

The funny thing is that vaping contains the same levels of nitrosamines that are found in medically approved nicotine patches.

Studies show that on average electronic cigarettes contain 8.18ng/g. Each ng is equal to one billionth of a gram (or millilitre (ml)); basically a minuscule level.

Compare that to a nicotine 4mg piece of gum, which contains 2ng/g, a nicotine 4mg patch which contains 8ng/g and a Marlboro US (full) which contains 11,960ng/g (err... WOW!); and you'll start to understand why there is no need for concern.

So... electronic cigarettes contain 1200 less nitrosamines than the levels found in tobacco cigarettes.

Vaping would NOT be any more likely to cause cancer than using nicotine gum or patches.

Before we move on, let me give you one important FACT about second hand vapour; as we know there are many that claim that vapour is just as dangerous as smoke from a tobacco cigarette.

Electronic cigarette vapour DOES NOT contain any cancer causing nitrosamines. However it does contain low levels of nicotine.

Now in enclosed spaces this can cause others around you to get a nicotine 'buzz', so I would take the same precautions when vaping around young children as I would if I were smoking.

Another possible side effect with second hand vapour is having an allergic reaction to Propylene Glycol (PG).

People allergic to PG will also be allergic to many common household products that also contain PG. So they may also develop an allergic reaction to the PG in the vapour you exhale (in closed spaces); however this is quite rare.

The best thing about vaping (and if you've stopped smoking) is that you can say goodbye to the 4000+ chemicals found in tobacco cigarettes.

Here are just a few:

- 1-aminonaphthalene - a carcinogen
- 2-aminonaphthalene - causes bladder cancer
- Acetone – ingredient in nail polish remover
- Ammonia – industrial cleaner and detergent
- Arsenic – lethal poison
- Benzene - causes several types of cancers
- Cadmium – used in batteries, a carcinogen
- Carbon monoxide – poisonous gas
- Cyanhydric acid – poisonous gas
- DDT – insecticide
- Dibenzacridine – a carcinogen
- Formaldehyde – embalming fluid
- Hydrogen Cyanide – weakens lungs
- Lead – a carcinogen
- Methanol – used as rocket fuel
- Naphthalene – moth repellent
- Naphthylamine – a carcinogen
- Nickel – a carcinogen
- Polonium 210 – a radioactive element
- Pyrene – a carcinogen
- Tar - contains several cancer-causing chemicals
- Vinyl Chloride – used in plastic materials

How to Vape

Vaping is really simple, but it's slightly different to smoking. The first time you vape it will feel very strange. You're use to smoke entering your lungs and taking 'hard drags'.

With vaping the trick is to take 'slow and steady' pulls.

It only takes a short amount of time to find your style of vaping and get use to manipulating the results.

For example if you want to see more vapour then you do not hold it in for as long. Or if you want to taste more flavour then you can exhale through your nose.

But the main thing that I want to point out is the type of pulls that you might take.

Mouth Pulls (Mouth hits)

This is the most common method. It's the way that smokers smoke as well. You pull the vapour into your mouth and then inhale. After a few seconds you exhale.

You won't produce as much vapour as you would from a direct pull, but you'll enjoy a more pleasant and satisfying vape, with no coughing, throat irritations or possible damage.

Direct Pulls (Lung hits)

Now this method is not so common. It's normally used by advanced vapers with mechanical mods and rebuildable atomisers when cloud chasing. If you want to get into cloud chasing you will need to learn how to do this technique.

Low nicotine strength e-liquid (below 6mg) with no menthol are very important to remain comfortable while doing these types of pulls. High nicotine levels can be harsh on your throat and cause you to cough; as well as cause irritation and/or possible damage.

When pulling from the drip tip (or mouthpiece) and inhaling (instead of filling your mouth then inhaling) you pull straight into your lungs. You breathe it in.

You will inhale and produce a lot more vapour than a mouth pull, but as stated you need to be careful with this type of pull. Due to the heat from the coil it can cause severe irritation or damage to your throat.

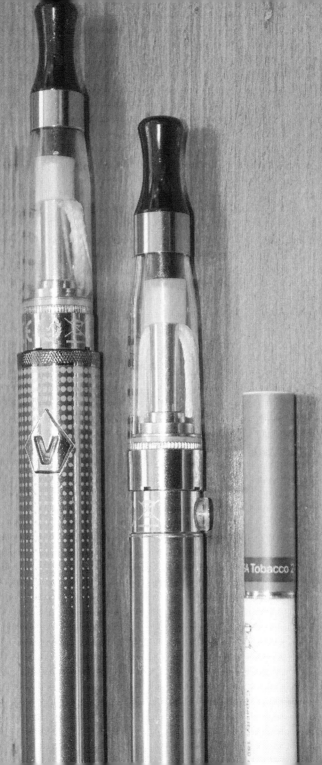

THE
ELECTRONIC
CIGARETTE

4 What is an Electronic Cigarette?

An e-cigarette is made up of two basic components. A charged battery and either a cartomiser, clearomiser or rebuildable atomiser filled with e-liquid.

Inside the cartomiser and clearomiser is a mini atomiser containing the heating element; the coil. Inside a rebuildable atomiser is just the coil.

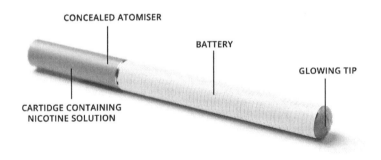

CONCEALED ATOMISER

BATTERY

GLOWING TIP

CARTIDGE CONTAINING
NICOTINE SOLUTION

The most important part of an electronic cigarette is the atomiser. The atomiser contains the coil (or coils) that heat up, from the power fed to it by the battery; and vaporise the e-liquid. You then inhale the vapour.

E-liquid is fed to the coils via wicks. Some wicks are long; some are short and can be made from different materials. Silica, stainless steel mesh and cotton are the main materials.

The coils ultimately affect the type of vape that you get. You will get either, a lot of vapour, flavour, throat hit and/or heat OR hardly any vapour, flavour, throat hit and/or heat.

You can read more about coils in 'Single & Dual Coils '.

Not all atomisers are the same; even though they are all made up of the same fundamental elements and serve the same purpose. They produce different results based on their design and the coils that are used.

5 Cig-a-likes

These small devices are designed to look like cigarettes. For new users they are the easiest (and most natural) to use when transitioning from tobacco cigarettes because of their size, look and feel.

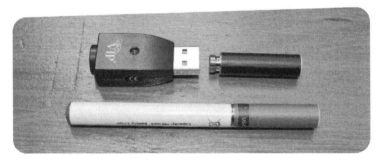

Most have a glowing tip that will light up when you inhale to simulate a tobacco cigarette and they come with either an automatic or manual battery.

With an automatic battery you simply take a pull and the battery will activate and you receive a small amount of vapour. With a manual battery you will need to push a button every time you take a pull.

There are two types of cig-a-likes.

Disposable

These are mainly found in petrol stations and shops. All of the basic components are enclosed in a cigarette looking plastic casing, so you will not be able to replace any parts, recharge or refill it. You simply throw it away when it stops working.

This type of electronic cigarette is not very reliable, so if you absolutely must buy a disposable, you should ensure that you buy from a reputable company.

Rechargeable

This type of electronic cigarette is the most popular; mainly because of its looks, simplicity and extendable length of use. They are made up of two parts, a rechargeable battery and a cartomiser.

You will also receive a USB charger for recharging the battery.

The cartomiser is prefilled with e-liquid that will last for a predetermined number of puffs. However you will normally see each cartomiser being advertised as the equivalent of 'X amount of cigarettes', normally forty.

You can buy them in many different flavours and nicotine strengths, so will have no problems with finding something that suits you.

When you notice that you are no longer getting any vapour, you simply throw the cartomiser away and replace it with a new one.

You may be able to refill it depending on the type that you have bought. If it has a removable top cap you can remove this and use a syringe to fill it. However these cartomisers do not hold much liquid, so take your time and refill it a few drops at a time.

So what's the conclusion?

They are lightweight, portable and less obvious. The battery charges quickly and they are good for reducing tobacco cigarette intake.

However, they are expensive and are not very effective if you want to quit smoking long term. Very little vapour is produced and the battery charge does not last for long.

They are definitely not suitable for heavy smokers; you'll find that you'll want to move on very quickly.

6 Pen Style Personal Vaporisers

Pen style devices are much larger than a cig-a-likes but this is the natural step up for those wanting a better vaping experience.

You can fill them with your own choice of e-liquid and the battery life is far superior to cig-a-likes. One charge can last you a whole day.

There are three main types of pen style devices.

Traditional Pen Style

These devices truly look like fancy, unusual pens or felt tip markers. With some them you could be easily fooled into picking it up in order to write something down.

They come in two parts... the battery and a matching cartomiser.

When you remove the lid you will find the mouth piece. Their size, inconspicuous designs and functionality make them very popular. You'll often see celebrities sporting these devices.

eGo Type

eGo style devices were the first mid-sized electronic cigarettes. They are very similar to traditional pen style devices but slightly thicker.

They are made up of one part... the battery. You will need to attach a cartomiser or clearomiser to the top of these batteries. Your choices with an eGo allow you to further customise your vaping experience.

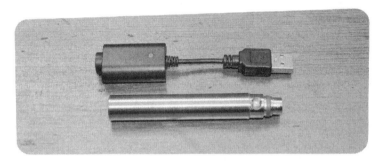

The eGo battery was invented by a company called Janty and manufactured by another company called Joyetech. The problem was that they did not patent their design and now there are many 'legal' clones of the original 'Joyetech eGo' design.

This level is where most people (including myself) start to have a more satisfying vaping experience. You'll notice instantly that you get a lot more flavour and vapour, mainly due to the cartomiser or clearomiser that you are able to attach.

They are available in many lengths. The shorter the length of the battery the shorter the battery life will be. Battery life is measured in mAh and mAh is explained later in this book.

To operate it, you will need to press a small button while you inhale, but you get use to this small requirement very quickly. Some eGo batteries will have USB ports at the bottom, allowing them to be used while they are being charged.

Variable Voltage Pen Style

There is the slightly larger ego type battery. They have a twist dial at the bottom that allows you to change the voltage (I explain more about this in sections 8 and 9).

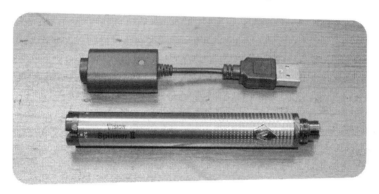

In a nutshell the higher the voltage, the more vapour produced. However you may lose some of the flavour and you could experience a burnt taste depending on the e-liquid that you use.

Or you may find that the flavour is slightly improved, especially with very sweet e-liquids. The lower the voltage the more flavour you will taste but less vapour is produced. It really does allow you to further customise the flavour and vapour to your own preferences over a standard eGo style battery.

There is also slightly more advanced devices available such as the iTaste VV. They are square, pen shaped. They are electrical with a microprocessor and a tiny screen. You push buttons as oppose to turning dials. The latest version comes with variable wattage as well as variable voltage, making it very similar to an electrical mod; but smaller.

So what's the conclusion?

Pen styles produce more vapour than cig-a-likes, are available with longer battery life and are available in more designs; such as metals like sleek stainless steel, beautiful solid colours, designer glitter and florescent multi coloured.

With variable voltage devices the batteries have higher mAh ratings so they can last two days or more depending on usage and you can customise your vaping more to your preferences. They are very safe due to their inbuilt safety features.

With the exception of the traditional pen style, the only negative is that they are more obvious.

7 Mods Adv. Personal Vaporisers

The ultimate vaping device!

Mods are the most customisable and powerful of all the electronic cigarette devices available. Although they are designed (and best suited) to be used with a rebuildable atomiser you do have the option of using clearomisers; if you don't want to get into coil building.

Mods are not batteries (like the eGo), but containers that hold replaceable and rechargeable batteries.

The best batteries to use in these devices are IMR and INR 'chemistry safe' batteries, so you can't just pop a Duracell in there. Although some people use ICR batteries in their mods, they are not recommended.

Unprotected ICR batteries should definitely not be used in mechanical mods as these have a greater risk of overheating. This can cause your battery to vent and possibly explode.

For full information on mods and rebuildable atomisers you should read volume two in this series.

Whether you decide to go for an electrical or mechanical mod you'll find that they both come in a variety of shapes and sizes (mainly tube and box styles) and the designs can be quite elaborate. In fact you could describe some of them as works of art; displaying intricate details carved into metal or wood.

There are two types of mods available; electrical mods and mechanical mods.

Electrical Mods

Electrical (or regulated) mods are fairly easy to use and contain a microprocessor that controls a number of safety features. Most electrical mods will include an ohm reader, made obvious by a small led screen on the side.

This can save you from having to purchase a separate ohm meter. An ohm reader is more commonly known as a resistance tester as a standalone device. Even if your mod does contain an ohm reader you may want to invest in a separate resistance tester for greater flexibility; especially if you are looking to build your own coils.

As well as having control over the voltage, you can also control the wattage on these devices. This aids in a more customisable and satisfactory vape. To understand how this works read section 9, 'Variable Wattage & Variable Voltage'.

Mechanical Mods

Mechanical mods are for serious vapers who are prepared to spend the time (and money) buying the right equipment, learning how to use them correctly and building coils. There really is no point of having a mechanical mod if you're not going to use rebuildable atomisers.

Notice that I did not state that they are for 'advanced vapers' but rather for 'serious vapers'. If you're willing to learn the basics (including safety precautions) it does not matter how long you've been vaping.

Mechanical mods are very complex and this section is not intended to provide full coverage of all of the various aspects.

A mechanical mod has electrical components whatsoever. When the firing button is engaged it completes a circuit that delivers unregulated current to your rebuildable atomiser.

So what's the conclusion?

Mods produce bigger clouds (vapour) and better flavour when paired with a good rebuildable atomiser. They are highly customisable, so you can combine pieces that are tailored to your personal style and preferences.

Mods are cheap to run and mechanical mods are extremely durable. Electrical mods provide a great deal of inbuilt protection making them **great devices for beginners**.

However, some mods can be heavy or bulky and initial costs can be expensive. They can be time consuming, as in order to get the best out of them you will need to build coils; and they will need cleaning.

With mechanical mods you will need to pay special attention to safety.

8 Understanding mAh, Voltage and Ohms

When purchasing equipment, there's a lot of numbers floating around that can be very confusing. The information here will give you a better understanding of what type of electronic cigarette (or personal vaporiser) to choose, to best suit your needs.

mAh

mAh refers to the battery life. Generally the lower the 'mAh' the smaller the size and life of the battery. For example a 650 mAh battery is approximately 70mm in length and a 1000 mAh battery is approximately 95mm in length.

100 mAh = approximately 1 hour

So a 650 mAh battery will last approximately 6.5 hours before it needs to be recharged. However, this will vary depending on how often you vape and the type of atomiser that you use.

- Cig-a-likes: available between 90 – 350 mAh
- Pen style: available between 650 – 1000 mAh.
- Variable Voltage Pen style: between 400 – 1600 mAh.

Batteries for mods are different. As stated earlier you will need to buy special batteries to put into a mod. Mod batteries also use mAh values and these typically range between 700 – 3500 mAh.

Voltage (Volts)

'Volts' refers to the power of the battery and it controls how hot the atomiser coil burns. The more volts they put out, the more vapour and flavour your atomiser can produce. However on variable voltage devices and electrical mods, if the voltage is set too high it may cause your e-liquid to taste burnt.

- Most Pen Style batteries run between 3.2 to 3.7 volts
- Variable Voltage batteries run between 3.3 to 4.8 volts

Mods are different. Electrical mods can run between 3 to 6 volts. But mechanical mods run on the natural voltage of the battery; so as the battery power drains the voltage decreases.

Ohms

'Ohms' refers to the measure of resistance to the electricity (power) that comes out of the battery. The term "ohm" is used when describing or selecting the coils inside rebuildable atomisers, clearomisers or cartomisers. Your coil inside your atomiser is built to a certain ohm rating.

A high resistance (1.2 ohm and upwards) coil offers a higher resistance to the electricity from the battery, which will result in less heat to the coil.

Most replaceable coils that come with more advanced clearomisers are only offered between 1.5 and 2.1 ohms. So the best way to get coils with a different ohm rating is to use a rebuildable atomiser and make it yourself.

New sub ohm replaceable coils have entered the market for a few brands of clearomisers which go as low as 0.8 ohms.

Low resistance coils (below 1.2 ohms) provide less resistance, therefore the coils get hotter, faster. Increased heat equals increased throat hit and vapour. However, low resistance coils draw more power from the battery.

All devices (with the exception of mechanical mods) have safety features built in and will not operate with low ohm coils.

9 Variable Wattage & Variable Voltage

So what is variable voltage and variable wattage? Well they both control the power provided to your atomiser. Most electrical mods come with variable voltage and variable wattage. Mechanical mods do not come with either.

What is Variable Voltage?

The best example I was given and can give to you, to explain variable voltage and variable wattage is as follows.

Imagine you're in a car. Your gas (accelerator) pedal is variable voltage and your cruise control is variable wattage. You want to maintain 50mph.

With your gas pedal, if you are going uphill you would need to press down to get to back up to 50mph.

And if you start to go downhill you would need to take your foot off the gas pedal otherwise you may find yourself going much faster than 50mph.

Variable voltage is a setting that you must manually adjust with each different circumstance. Your different rebuildable atomisers or clearomisers and the coils inside are the changing road conditions.

Now in order for you to find your 'sweet spot' on a variable voltage device you would start at the lowest voltage and work your way up until the vape you experience (the flavour, throat hit, vapour and heat) is just right for you.

What is Variable Wattage?

Well variable wattage is a 'set it and leave it' control. Just like cruise control in a car.

For example, let's say you've been vaping using variable voltage and found your 'sweet spot' at **4.3 volts** for a particular e-liquid. And you know that the coil inside your attached clearomiser or rebuildable atomiser has an ohm resistance of **2.1 ohms**.

Now if you only intend on using variable voltage then you're happy to press or release the gas pedal every now and then.

But if you use variable wattage you'll have fewer adjustments to make. In fact you'll only have to set your level once.

Going back to our example:

> *When you turn on your cruise control in your car you would simply set it to 50mph and regardless of the road condition you will maintain a consistent 50mph.*

Variable wattage will give you a consistent vape regardless of what type of rebuildable atomiser or clearomiser you attach to your device.

To work out what figure you would need to set the variable wattage on your device to you will need to do some basic math. We'll use the figures highlighted above.

Watts = (Volts x Volts) / Ohms

So our calculation will be:

(4.3 x 4.3) / 2.1 = 8.80

Or

18.49 / 2.1 = 8.80

You can also go online and use a 'variable wattage calculator' or an 'ohms law' calculator.

After entering 4.3 volts and 2.1 ohms into a calculator, it will give you a wattage calculation of 9 watts (or 8.80 to be precise).

You can then set your device to 9 watts. Now, no matter what clearomiser or rebuildable atomiser you attach to your device you will still achieve your 'sweet spot'.

How does it do this?

Your variable wattage device uses an inbuilt microprocessor and automatically reads the ohm resistance of your clearomiser or rebuildable atomiser and makes automatic adjustments to the voltage.

Let's say you attach a different clearomiser with a coil resistance of 1.8ohms. Your device will still be at 9 watts, but it will read that the ohm resistance is now 1.8ohms and automatically adjust the voltage (to around 4 volts).

The beauty is that you don't even have to worry about how it does the calculations. Just let it 'do its thing'.

Choices!

Some people prefer variable voltage to variable wattage, and in most cases it boils down to the level of control you want when vaping.

Coil ohm (resistance) levels can fluctuate slightly. So your coil might read 2.1ohms at the start and then a week later read 1.8ohms.The advantage of variable wattage is that you don't have to worry about checking your coil ohms and making manual adjustments.

Variable wattage is ideal if you use a lot of different clearomisers and rebuildable atomisers. Variable voltage is good if you only use one clearomiser or rebuildable atomiser and you are willing to make minor adjustments to the voltage.

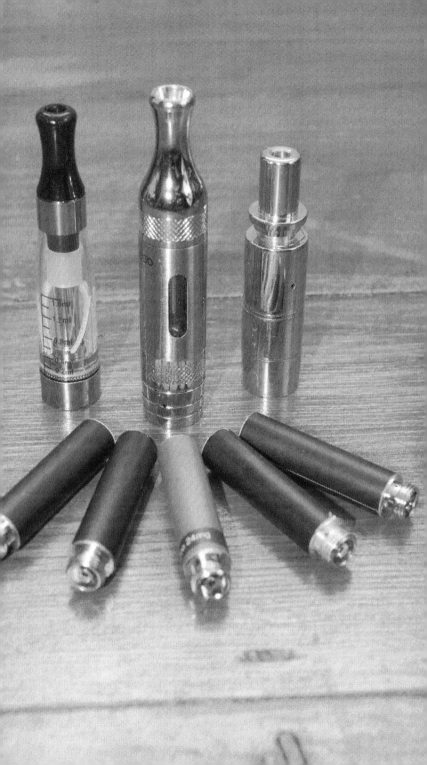

CARTOMISERS CLEAROMISERS & RBAs

10 Cartomisers

The first electronic cigarettes were made up of three parts; a small battery, atomiser and cartridge. However they were prone to leaking. A solution was found by combining the atomiser and cartridge. This was the birth of the Cartomiser

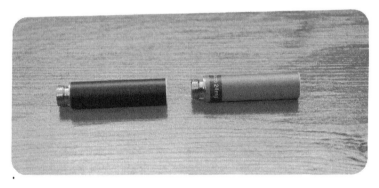

A cartomiser is the section that looks like the filter section of a tobacco cigarette; although they come in various colours, not just tan.

Inside a cartomiser is a tiny coil that is surrounded by a polyfill material. This polyfill material is soaked in e-liquid. When you take a puff the battery activates, heating the coil and the coil heats up the liquid which mixes with the air taken in. The e-liquid is vaporised and you inhale the result... the vapour.

You can buy blank cartomisers that you can fill with your own e-liquid and attach to an eGo battery. They tend to come with very high ohm coils, typically 2.4 – 2.8 ohms; but you can find lower. Due to their small size they can only hold a small amount of e-liquid; typically 1ml.

Some cartomisers come in a 510 size which allows you to use your own drip tip; simply remove the plastic insert and slot in the drip tip of your choice.

You can also buy the prefilled cartomisers. Each cartomiser is meant to contain enough puffs to equal approximately 20-40 cigarettes; the different manufacturers will make different statements. These cartomisers are built to be disposable. However people often refill them a few times before throwing them away.

For some people cartomisers are not satisfying and they quickly migrate to clearomisers. However, cartomisers are still in wide use.

Some people love the look, especially when going out as they are less obvious. Others attach the prefilled cartomisers to better batteries (with the use of thread adapters) and some people even use them as dripping devices for testing their DIY e-liquid.

11 Clearomisers

Before the invention of clearomisers, vapers would experience 'dry hits' or 'run out' unexpectedly, as they were unable to see when their cartomiser needed to be refilled.

The idea then came of being able to see what was inside... from the outside. After some development, they started to make cartomisers out of thin, clear plastic.

The first clearomisers were not the best choice, but because of the benefits people continued to use them.

This lead to manufacturers constantly developing and greatly improving clearomisers; which now out sell cartomisers around the world. In fact nearly all starter kits will include a clearomiser or two.

Clearomisers are a very popular choice!

Plastic, glass, mini, large, disposable, reusable and some coils are even rebuildable (even though they are not designed to be rebuilt, you'll need to know what you are doing and use an ohm meter).

There are replaceable parts for all but the very basic models. You can replace the coils, the mouthpieces (or drip tips with some) and even the tanks.

Something to look out for is 'flooding'. If you hear a gurgling sound when you take a pull on your clearomiser, it has probably flooded. Not a problem... it means that you have accidently allowed e-liquid to drop into the centre channel.

To fix this problem, simply remove the clearomiser from the battery and blow firmly into the mouthpiece to push the excess e-liquid out. Hold a paper towel under the threaded end.

Top Coil Clearomisers

In this type of clearomiser, the coil is at the top of the tank. There are long wicks which hang down into the tank. The wicks draw liquid up towards the coil and the coil vaporises the liquid.

When the liquid falls below the reach of the wicks you will need to refill. Or you can 'tip and spin' to coat the wicks with whatever liquid is left inside the tank.

The main disadvantage is that if you want to change flavours you will need to either wash it (and let it dry) or change to another clearomiser. This is because the long wicks hold a lot of liquid and can hold it for a very long time.

You may also experience a plastic taste, due to the coil being at the top and heating the plastic mouthpiece while vaping, but in general it is not problem.

These clearomisers are made of plastic and although popular they are not designed to last for a long time; but thankfully they are fairly cheap to replace. They are also not the best looking devices; an example would be the CE4 clearomiser.

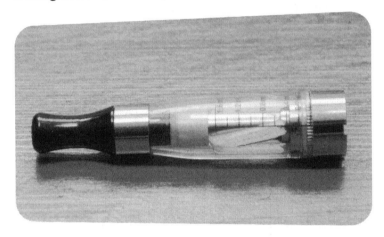

The good news is that it is very rare for them to leak.

To fill you simply take off the mouthpiece and pour the liquid in from the top. Wait for about ten minutes to let the wicks become saturated, then vape. As the coils are at the top, the vape is normally warm and the throat hit much stronger.

Bottom Coil Clearomisers

In order to combat the wicking issues associated with top coil clearomisers the bottom coil clearomiser was created.

Instead of having the coil at the top and the long wicks drawing the liquid upwards, the coil is situated at the bottom and the clearomiser uses gravity and a vacuum seal to feed the e-liquid to the much smaller wicks inside the coil unit at the bottom. The only disadvantage is that if the vacuum seal fails you can get small leaks.

To fill these clearomisers you need to turn the unit upside down. Fiddly at first but you get use to it. The vape is normally much smoother and cooler than with a top coil clearomiser.

The flavour with these devices is also better than top coil clearomisers and it is much easier to change flavours. So you won't need to wash and dry it so often.

This is because the small wicks inside the coil unit do not hold much liquid, so you can simply refill and after a few puffs the new flavour will come through.

A good example would be the Innokin iClear 30.

Glassomisers

Glassomisers are bottom coil clearomisers with one main difference. The tanks are made of glass rather than plastic, so they can last a lot longer than clearomisers.

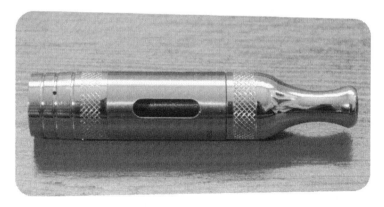

There are many e-liquids that contain flavourings (such as cinnamon) and citrus extracts which are known as 'tank crackers'. These ingredients can basically melt certain plastic tanks. Hence using a glassomiser is often the better choice, even if they are more expensive.

The tanks are made from Pyrex glass which means that they are completely resistant to erosion. So regardless of what ingredients are in your e-liquid, your tank will never melt. This is covered in the e-liquid section.

Some people believe that using a glassomiser improves the taste of your e-liquid. I would have to agree, although it's not a 'mind blowing' difference.

You will be spoilt for choice when choosing a glassomiser. I believe that the extra expense is worth it; especially due to the higher build quality, durability and not having to worry about what you put in it. An example would be the Aspire ET-S (although at the time of writing there are manufacturing issues with their replacement coils).

The only disadvantage is that the tanks are prone to break if dropped or put under pressure (i.e. squashed in your pocket). I have never experienced a broken tank; so (as with anything made of glass) if you look after your glassomiser you'll be fine. Plus you can buy replacement glass tanks for a fraction of the cost of replacing the whole glassomiser.

12 Rebuildable Atomisers (RBAs)

Rebuildable atomisers are exactly that. You build the coils that are inside.

You can tweak them to exactly how you want. Choose the ohms of the coils, the gauge of wire and choose the type of wick you want. They provide the best flavour, the most amount of vapour and (once you have paid for your RBA or RDA) they are the cheapest to run.

The common myth is that you can only use rebuildable atomisers on mechanical mods, but that is not true. As long as you keep to a single coil build (over 1.8 ohms) you can use a rebuildable atomiser on an ego style battery; variable voltage or not.

If you do use them with a mod then there are a lot more options (in terms of coil building) available to you.

You can get single coil RBAs, dual coil RBAs and even quad coil RBAs that allow you to have four coils. There's a whole world of rebuildable atomisers out there.

Now if you are not into fiddling or just want to vape and go, rebuildable atomisers are not for you. As in order for them to function you will need to keep building coils periodically.

It takes some time and practice. But once you've got it nailed you may never want to go back to clearomisers again. For a more comprehensive look at rebuildable atomisers, take a look at volume 2.

There are two types of RBAs.

Rebuildable Tank Atomisers (RTAs)

These come with a tank to store your e-liquid. You simply build your coil, fit your wick and then re-attach the tank and drip tip.

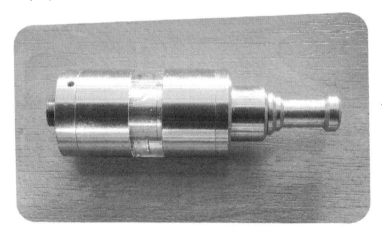

The flavour is good and due to the tank you can vape away for hours or even days; depending on the size of the tank and how often you vape.

Rebuildable Dripping Atomisers (RDAs)

These are not built with a tank. You build your coil as normal, install it; add your wicking material applying a small amount of e-liquid.

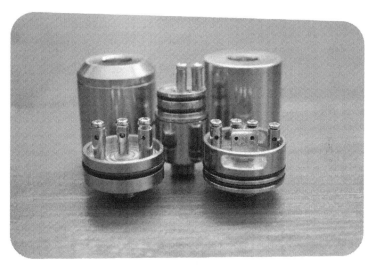

You then put the cover on and then drop e-liquid onto your wick every 5-10 puffs; depending on when you taste the flavour diminishing or when you start to get a dry hit.

You e-liquid can taste completely different in and RDA. They produce great flavour but the only disadvantage is that you have to keep topping it up.

13 Single & Dual Coils

You should now have a good idea as to how RBAs, clearomisers and cartomisers work; and the fact that the engine in all of these devices is the coil.

Not everyone is interested in talking about coils, but it is the most important part of your electronic cigarette. And you'll understand why shortly.

All devices will have at least one coil (single), some will have two (dual) and you can buy RBAs that allow you to set up four coils (quad). I've seen some pretty creative coil builds using eight coils and I'm sure that someone has used more; but we won't focus on that.

Now the beauty about electronic cigarettes is that there are so many devices and options available that if you don't want to get into building coil, you don't have to.

You can buy a clearomiser with inbuilt coils or for a better experience you can buy clearomisers that use replaceable coil units that are available as single or dual coil configurations. You just screw one in and when it starts to taste burnt (after a week or two) you swap it for another. Job done!

But if you want to understand how coils affect your vaping experience... read on!

So what's the difference?

In this section we'll look at each one individually; so that you can make an informed decision when purchasing or building your own coils.

However, nothing quite beats trying a single coil set up next to a dual coil set up and actually seeing, and tasting the differences.

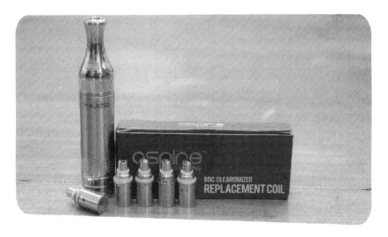

So why have more than one coil?

Well basically, each coil adds more heat and the extra heat from two or four coils will either double or quadruple the heat and vapour production. The more heat produced, the stronger the flavour and the warmer and more luxurious the vapour clouds. Something for you to note is that not everyone likes a 'hot vape' and some e-liquids can taste burnt at high temperatures.

Single Coil Builds

Single coil builds consume less battery power as they only need power to drive one coil. They also consume less e-liquid, as only one coil is in contact with the e-liquid.

The biggest advantage of single coil builds is that they are easier to build and less time consuming. Unfortunately single coil builds do not produce as much vapour, but it still may be adequate for your needs.

Dual Coil Builds

The biggest advantage of dual coil builds is that they produce a superior amount of vapour (due to there being more heat). Unfortunately because there are more coils your battery will drain much faster than with a single coil build as dual coils need more power.

Also with two coils now in contact with the e-liquid you will find that you'll consume much larger amounts of e-liquid (there has to be a consequence of producing all of that thick rich vapour). Finally the most obvious disadvantage is that they are harder to build, which means that they can be time consuming.

Single and dual coil comparison

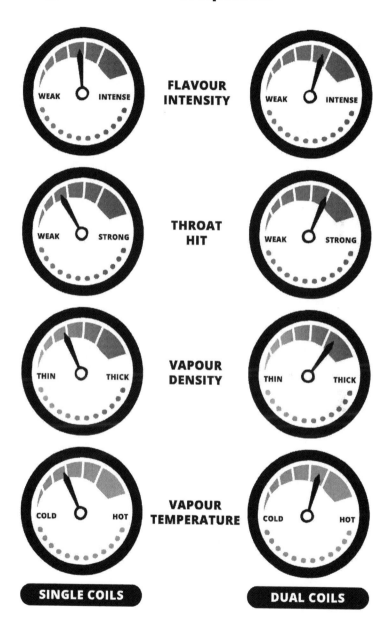

FLAVOUR INTENSITY

THROAT HIT

VAPOUR DENSITY

VAPOUR TEMPERATURE

SINGLE COILS

DUAL COILS

Having more control over your vape

Ok! So we know that the coil is the element that heats up when the battery is activated; causing the e-liquid to also heat up and vaporise. And that it is the main element that controls flavour, vapour production and more.

But what if that coil was built in a 'sloppy' manner and causes your e-liquid to taste funny or even worse... stops working.

Not a big deal if you buy premade coil units or clearomisers with inbuilt coils. You simply swap it for another. However these units can be expensive and the cost can add up over time. You are also limited by the ohm rating of the coil units available; typically between 1.5 ohms and 2.1 ohms.

I'm not going to cover ohms or resistance in this volume as you won't need to worry about this if you are only buying devices with inbuilt or replaceable coil units.

However, the only way to completely control your vaping experience is to build your own coils!

This is where RBAs start to shine. There is a short learning curve but the rewards are worth the effort. You'll also save a lot of money. If you competently build and install a coil, it can last a maximum of six months. Yes... six months!

Ok... let's get real!

This would be true if you're a very, very light vaper. And even if you are a light vaper, the eventual build-up of burnt e-liquid stuck to the coil would seriously affect the taste.

And no matter how much you try to clean that coil you will never get it as good as new. Quick note... we're talking about the rebuildable setups where you build the coil first, then put in the wick.

The average life expectancy of this type of coil when used by an average vaper is two to four weeks. On average I'll build a new coil every seven to fourteen days.

A ten metre length of resistance wire can make approximately one hundred coils and costs around £5 ($8). And a bag of organic cotton wool will last at least a year, costing around £4 ($6).

You will have to buy an RBA, but they last years and the running cost per year (from the figures above) is approximately £9 ($14). You can build lower ohm coils (e.g. 1.4ohms) which will produce more vapour and flavour.

The choice is yours! But you can see the attraction.

But let's face it... not everyone wants to start fiddling with bits of wire and cotton wool.

14 Filling Your Device

Filling up is very easy for most devices.

RTAs come with a fill hole within the base. You would simply remove the screw and fill up the tank. Due to their 'vacuum seal' design they can be fiddly (vol.2 goes into more detail).

Filling a cartomiser

Remove the plastic insert from the top of the cartomiser. You will notice a soft gauze type material inside. Cartomiser are not transparent and hold very little e-liquid (around 1 ml) so you will need to fill in intervals. Place the nozzle of your bottle inside the tube and squeeze gently. As you squeeze rotate the cartomiser.

Once you see liquid starting to gather at the top stop filling and allow the liquid to sink in. Repeat until the liquid no longer soaks in and stays wet at the top. This method is time consuming. Using a syringe (with needle) is much quicker.

Once you have filled your cartomiser, replace the plastic insert and blow into it to remove any e-liquid that may have found its way into the small opening by the bottom threads.

Filling a clearomiser or glassomiser

Each device will have an indicator showing the maximum level that the unit should be filled. Filling beyond this point can cause problems (such as flooding). If your device does not have an indicator, it is best to only fill the unit up to 75%.

Before you fill up, look into your clearomiser; you will see a small vertical tube. Try not to get any e-liquid in this tube. If you do, your device may flood, causing it to flood.

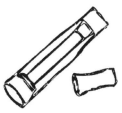

Step 1 - Prepare
Remove the mouthpiece from the top of your clearomiser and hold it at a 45 degree angle.

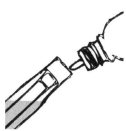

Step 2 – Fill it up
Place the nozzle of your e-liquid bottle against the inside of your clearomiser and fill slowly up to the fill line.

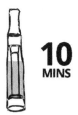

Step 3 – Let it rest
Replace the mouthpiece and allow adequate time for the e-liquid to soak into the wick. The recommended time is ten minutes, but if you're refilling with the same e-liquid it can be less.

For more advanced clearomisers and glassomisers you will need to fill from the bottom. The process is the same except you turn the unit upside down and remove the section at the bottom (that holds the coil unit). You can then fill your device.

15 Priming Your Device

You've filled your cartomiser, clearomiser or RTA... you're excited. You start vaping. But then you notice a burnt taste.

That can't be right!

Well what has most likely happened is that the coil in your device has not been properly primed.

What is priming?

Your device contains a coil and wick. You fill your device with e-liquid which then soaks into the wick. When you activate your electronic cigarette the coil heats up and that heat burns the e-liquid in the wick.

If there is not sufficient e-liquid in the wick (it is dry) the wick will burn. This is what produces the burnt taste, which is hard to remove; once your wick is burnt it will not function properly again. With an RTA you can easily change your wick, but with other devices you may need to replace the whole device or coil unit.

Priming is ensuring that your wick has been sufficiently soaked in e-liquid.

Priming your device before use

After you've filled your device (with a sufficient amount of liquid) you should always wait <u>at least</u> ten minutes before vaping, with your device held in an upright position. This is so that the e-liquid can soak into the wick.

It is recommended that you wait ten - thirty minutes before use; especially when using thicker, high percentage Vegetable Glycerine (VG) e-liquids. Cartomisers and clearomisers are not suited for high VG e-liquids.

> *Sometimes you may notice a gurgling, 'slurpy' sound when taking a pull. Simply remove your device from the battery (or mod) and blow sharply through the mouthpiece. This will remove any excess liquid that may have found its way into the centre tube. You'll need some tissue to catch the excess liquid that comes out.*

Not filling up with enough e-liquid in a device that has not been used and is dry can also lead to a burnt wick.

Priming your device after use

If you've allowed sufficient time for your e-liquid to soak in but you are getting a burnt taste or dry hits, there may be trapped air which is not allowing the e-liquid to flow freely. You will need to prime your device in a different way.

Remove it from the battery (or mod). Cover the air hole with your finger and then take a short, sharp pull via the mouthpiece.

If you've blocked the air hole properly you should not be able to suck in any air. 1-2 times is enough; as anymore may cause your device to flood and gurgle causing you to have to blow out any excess liquid.

If priming and blowing out does not fix your device then something else is wrong; you may have a faulty coil.

Avoiding the dreaded burnt taste

1. **Don't pull for too long**
   The coil will remain active and you may overheat your e-liquid. Certain flavours can handle a long deep pulls (tobacco, menthol, coffee) but other e-liquids may taste better with a shorter deep pulls (fruity, sweet flavours).

2. **Take your time**
   Stop for a few seconds between pulls to allow your device to cool down and for the wick to draw in more liquid.

3. **Try not to flood your device**
   Your device may overwork in order to vaporise the excess liquid.

4. **Refill your device**
   Refilling your device before your e-liquid runs out will avoid getting a burnt taste.

Dry hits

A device that has not been properly primed or that has an insufficient amount of e-liquid remaining can lead to dry hits. A dry hit will cause irritation to your throat. You can use the 'priming your device after use' method to irradiate this.

16 Cleaning Your Devices

Your RBA, clearomiser and coils may become dirty or clogged due to the ingredients within e-liquids that accumulate inside your devices as the e-liquid is vaporised.

Some e-liquid flavours can be more problematic than others, but as a general rule the darker the e-liquid, the more likely it is that it will quickly dirty or clog your devices; much more quickly than a clearer liquid.

It's important to note that cleaning can extend the life of your devices and restore performance.

There are several signs that let you know that your device may need cleaning:

- Reduced vapour production
- No vapour production
- Difficulty drawing air through the device
- Burnt or harsh taste when using the device

If you experience reduced vapour production (or no vapour at all) you should check your battery first.

Ensure that it is fully charged and that the connections are clean. If the battery is working then it may be your coil that is faulty.

If cleaning your unit does not resolve the problem swap your device for another (if your coil is not replaceable). If your coil is replaceable change the coil unit or build another coil for your RBA.

The most common cleaning methods

1. Blowing it out (first step)

Just as you would for flooding, remove your device from the battery, place your lips on the mouthpiece or drip tip and blow firmly to force out the excess liquid or gunk onto a paper towel.

2. Hot water rinse (minor problems)

Place your device under hot water. Let it cool then blow it out to remove excess water. Set it an upright position and allow it to dry for 24 hours.

3. Soaking (recommended)

Soak your device in water for at least 30-60 minutes. Then blow it out to remove the excess water.

Soak it in water for a second time for at least 2-3 hours. Then blow it out to remove the excess water. Set it in an upright position and allow it to dry for 24 hours.

Note that some people use vodka instead of water and a few people will leave it to soak in vodka overnight for extreme problems. Vodka should be used as a last resort; drink it, don't waste it.

Don't forget your batteries

Whether you're using an eGo or variable voltage battery, an electrical or mechanical mod; e-liquid will find its way into your battery connections, which can reduce the flow of electricity to your attached device; affecting performance.

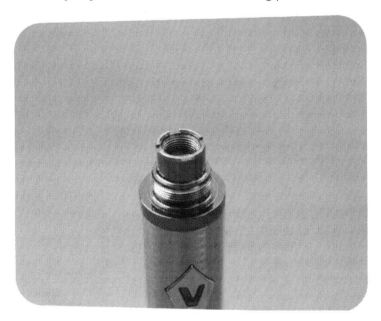

EGo and variable voltage batteries

Every two weeks (or if your battery needs cleaning now) take a cotton tip/swab (like a Q-tip) and gently remove the excess liquid. You can also apply a small amount of rubbing alcohol to the swab for a better clean.

Be gentle! Don't push on the centre connection.

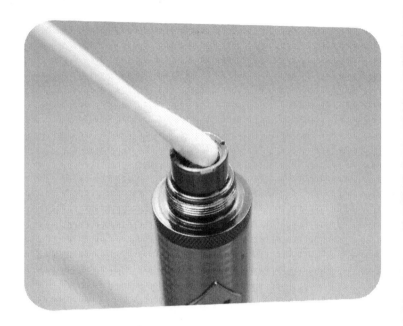

You will be surprised at the amount of dirt that collects in that area. For hard to reach places, you can use a toothpick or small cleaning brush.

Electrical and mechanical mods

As these devices have removable batteries, you will need to clean the mod itself; as opposed to the battery. This will require taken the unit apart in order to clean it properly. However as a temporary measure you can use the same method of using a cotton swab.

For more detailed information on mods, read volume 2.

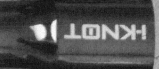

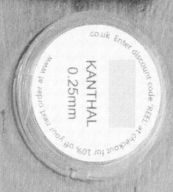

KANTHAL
0.25mm

co.uk Enter discount code 'REEL' at checkout for 10% off your next order at www.

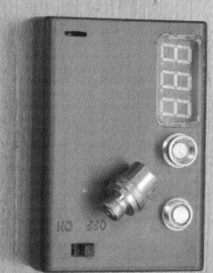

OFF ON

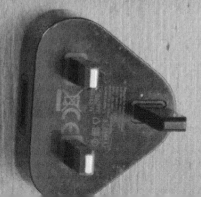

ACCESSORIES

17 USB Chargers

Most electronic cigarettes will come with a USB charger. If not you can buy one quite cheaply. You simply screw your battery into one end and push the USB end into a USB port on your laptop or computer.

If you don't have any spare USB ports or access to a laptop or computer you can add a USB wall charger. You screw the battery in as normal and then connect the end that would go into your computer's USB port into the USB wall charger. The charger is then plugged into the wall.

If you are on the move you can substitute the wall charger for a car charger (ensure that your car charger has a 1000mAh socket).

Never leave batteries unattended whilst charging!

18 Beauty Rings

This accessory also goes by several other names such as a vanity ring, cone adapter or plinth.

Clearomisers, RBAs or cartomisers will be manufactured with either a 510 or eGo connection. An eGo battery will accept both 'eGo' and '510' threaded clearomisers, RBAs or cartomisers.

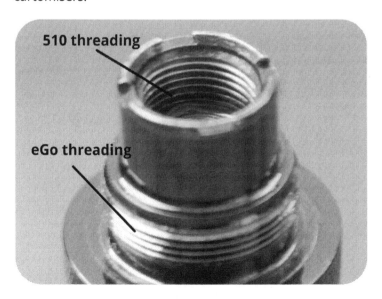

510 threading

eGo threading

If your clearomiser, RBA or cartomiser has an eGo threading it will have a 'female skirt' connection which overhangs when attached to the battery, covering all of the threads of an eGo battery.

But if your clearomiser, RBA or cartomiser has a 510 connection, you will still be able to see where the battery and your device connect.

A beauty ring will have eGo threading and simply covers the gap when connecting your device to an eGo battery.

Cylindrical Beauty Ring

This accessory screws onto your ego battery in order to hide the connection point, giving your electronic cigarette a much smoother look.

The cylindrical ring is good to use with smaller width clearomisers, RBAs and cartomisers (i.e. mini Vivi Nova tanks) that have the 510 threading that will not cover the outside threads of your eGo battery.

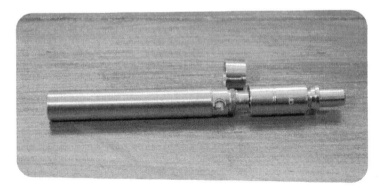

Shown above is an eGo battery without the beauty ring. Shown next is an eGo battery with a cylindrical beauty ring.

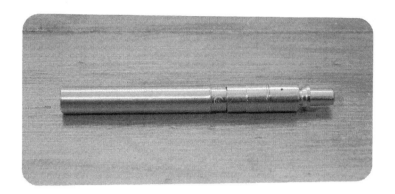

Flared Beauty Ring

This accessory also screws onto your ego battery in order to hide the eGo threads of the battery, to give your electronic cigarette a much smoother look.

The widening flare on this ring makes it ideal for use with larger clearomisers, RBAs and cartomisers (i.e. the 3.5ml Vivi Nova).

19 Drip Tips

These are small accessories that are used with rebuildable atomisers and some clearomisers. They are used in place of a fixed mouthpiece (like you would find on a CE4 clearomiser) and are normally pushed into place.

The most common drip tip size is '510' and they can be found with small openings (good for use with tanks) or with large openings where you can drip e-liquid directly onto the coil; good for RDAs (dripping atomisers).

Drip tips are used to improve the look of your electronic cigarette or for added comfort and they come in a very wide variety of shapes, sizes and materials. They can also affect the outcome of your vape, so try not to overlook the importance of them.

The smaller the opening the better the flavour tends to be and drip tips with wider openings allow you to inhale more vapour. You need to buy a few different styles and see how it changes your vape.

Another important feature of drip tips is that they create a safe distance between you and the heat from your atomiser as well as keeping e-liquid away from your lips. A drip tip is effectively a safety device in itself.

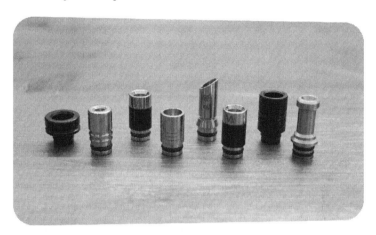

If you find that your existing drip tip is getting too hot you can buy a heat resistant drip tip or a drip tip insulator (as shown on the far left) to protect against burning lips.

Materials like Delrin, Pyrex, acrylic and ceramics help prevent heat transfer; or you can simply opt to use a longer drip tip.

Propylene glycol (PG) does have some anti-bacterial and anti-fungal properties, but you should clean your drip tips regularly to avoid any build-up.

You can clean your drip tips in hot, soapy water or alcohol to remove gunk and keep them germ-free. Note that alcohol can cause damage to acrylic drip tips if left in too long.

20 Other Accessories

You'll find a whole host of other non-essential accessories available for your devices. Here are a few of the items you will come across.

1. Electronic cigarette stands

2. Carry cases

3. Lanyards (from plain to glitter)

4. Metallic e-liquid holders

5. Electronic cigarette wraps (personalise your device)

If you're getting into rebuildable atomisers then you'll need several more items such as resistance wire and a resistance tester to name a few.

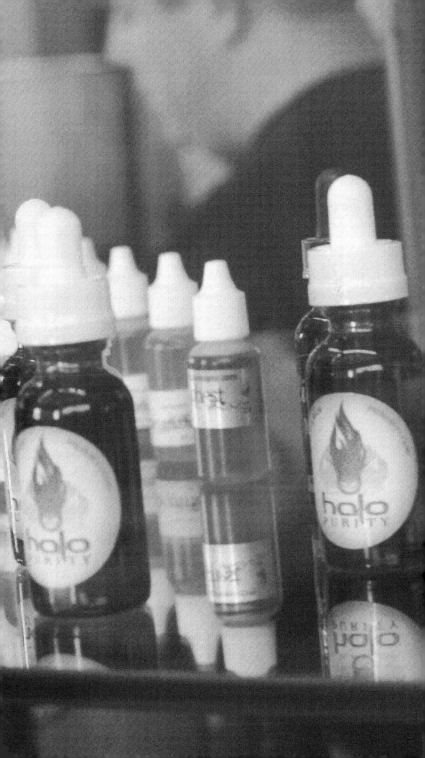

E-LIQUID

21 What is E-liquid?

E-liquid is the coal for your fire!

No matter what electronic cigarette you choose you will need e-liquid; whether you choose to buy or make it yourself.

E-liquid (or e-juice) comes in a wide variety of flavours ranging from simple one to two flavour liquids to complex recipes with three or more combined flavours.

Complex recipes are often referred to as 'gourmet' e-liquids; which are not your standard simple e-liquids. They will have a unique taste. It may have taken the creator months or years to perfect the recipe and when supplied to you they are normally ready to vape.

If you buy 'gourmet' e-liquid you will be hard pressed to distinguish all of the flavours due to the complexity of the vendor's recipe.

E-liquid evaporates when heated by the coil in your atomiser, producing flavoured vapour that you inhale.

It is made up of between two to five ingredients; unlike tobacco cigarettes which contain 4000+ ingredients.

The four main ingredients are:

- Nicotine
- Flavouring
- Propylene Glycol (PG)
- Vegetable Glycerine (VG)

Note that distilled water is sometimes used but not necessary. If it is used, it's used as a diluting agent (thinner) and some people will use vodka instead of distilled water.

To use e-liquid, you simply fill your tank, whether it be a cartomiser, clearomiser or rebuildable atomiser (RBAs). With dripping atomisers (RDAs) you would apply e-liquid every few puffs.

Don't let your eyes fool you!

E-liquids vary in terms of colour and thickness depending on the ingredients included. High nicotine juices tend to be darker in colour and high Vegetable Glycerine (VG) e-liquids will be thicker.

Definitely don't buy e-liquid because of its colour. Red, blue green etc. are NOT natural colours for e-liquid; even though they do look nice. And e-liquids containing high levels of VG can clog up, or be very hard to vape in, your more basic devices like cartomisers and top coil clearomisers.

22 Choosing Your Nicotine Strength

Nicotine in its pure form is a deadly toxic substance and should never be purchased or handled in a non-diluted state.

However, if purchased in a diluted form (premixed) it is perfectly safe to handle even in the case of a spill or skin contact; however you should keep it away from children and pets. Any e-liquid you that you do not make yourself can be regarded as premixed.

You would not normally be involved with high level liquid nicotine unless you get into DIY e-liquid mixing.

Nicotine strengths can be quite confusing at first but it is quite simple once you get the basic understanding. Some standard strengths of nicotine in e-liquids that you buy are:

3mg, 6mg, 12mg, 18mg, 24mg and 36mg.

The higher the mg level, the higher the nicotine content. The mg is <u>not</u> the amount that is in the bottle but the amount of nicotine in milligrams for each millilitre of e-liquid.

You may see a vendor express 12mg as 1.2%, but they both represent the same level of nicotine.

When choosing your nicotine strength it really is a case of 'trial and error, but you can use the following as a starting guide:

- 6mg is the equivalent of a very light cigarette
- 12mg is the equivalent of a medium cigarette
- 18mg is the equivalent of a normal cigarette
- 24mg is the equivalent of a heavy cigarette

Now not all of the nicotine in your e-liquid will be absorbed by your body, especially if you're a new vaper; as there are many factors that affect the absorption rate. In fact you may only end up taking in only 50% of the stated nicotine level.

The main reason is that as a new vaper you will be use to taking shorts pulls from a cigarette and this means you'll absorb less nicotine when using an electronic cigarette and vaping the same way you smoked.

Experienced vapers take long, slow pulls and can therefore absorb more nicotine from the same e-liquid and equipment as the new vaper.

Now... no electronic cigarette (even mods) can replicate the same level of nicotine absorption as a tobacco cigarette. So your cravings will be satisfied but you will be absorbing less nicotine.

So experienced vapers will lower their nicotine level as their body naturally becomes use to the lower nicotine absorption and they progress onto more efficient equipment.

So finding the right nicotine level is not just about finding the right mg level but also about your technique and equipment.

One word of caution is that if you set the nicotine strength too low and your body is still asking for more; you will find that you will vape a lot more. The last thing you want is to go out for the evening and have to constantly vape like a chimney just to feel satisfied.

If you are a new vaper it is advisable that you start at 12mg and above.

If you want to stay away from nicotine altogether but still crave the 'hand to mouth' action you can buy e-liquid that contains zero nicotine; which is becoming more and more popular as people try to break their dependency on nicotine.

I use to smoke 10-15 cigarettes a day and started on 18mg, but I found this too strong to use all day. But as a new non-smoker I still needed that nicotine kick in the mornings. So in the mornings I would use the 18mg and for the rest of the day I used a 12mg e-liquid.

As at the time of writing this I use 6mg all day and 3mg if I'm using an RDA (dripping atomiser). But you can use any combination of strengths you wish.

A word of warning!

Liquid nicotine is a highly addictive and toxic substance. If misused or mishandled it can lead to dangerous results. Do not leave any e-liquid where it can be reached by children, pets, or handled by individuals who are not capable of understanding its potential danger. Store and use your e liquid carefully and securely.

23 Choosing E-liquid

Now that you know a little more about e-liquid and its ingredients, you'll want to start trying some.

Keep it small!

If you are new to vaping or choosing new flavours you should buy your e-liquid in small sizes. Don't make the same mistake that I made. I bought 30ml bottles without knowing if I liked the taste and ended up throwing away several bottles.

Plus I knew nothing about steeping (explained later), which would have improved the flavour.

Experimenting with e-liquid can be expensive so look out for sample packs that allow you to try several different flavours; although they will come in smaller sizes (i.e. 1ml, 3ml or 5ml per flavour).

Don't colour my juice!

As stated before, don't buy e-liquid simply based on looks. Uncoloured e-liquids tend to range from clear to orangey brown to dark brown.

If it is blue, green, purple or any other colour that DOES NOT fall within the clear, tan, to brown spectrum I would steer clear, as it would indicate that it has been coloured.

If in doubt...ask!

Food colouring in your food is completely different from having food colouring in your e-liquid, which is completely unnecessary.

Yes! It may look nice, but think about your lungs!

Variety is the spice of ~~life~~ vaping!

Buy at least three or four different types of flavours to start with (dessert, fruit, tobacco, drinks).

Once you have identified which types of flavours you like the best, you can start buying e-liquid in that flavour range that suit your taste and large bottles of the flavours you really like.

I started by buying ONLY tobacco flavours. Big mistake for me! Now (after I broadened my horizons) I know that I like drink flavours (rum, coke, Irish cream, coffee and cocktails).

Experiment with your choices. If you were a menthol smoker, choose an e-liquid that has menthol. If you have a sweet tooth, try some of the candy flavours.

Just don't limit yourself to tobacco flavours. You'll find that none of them actually taste like a real cigarette, but some e-liquid makers are getting VERY close to replicating the taste.

You can also mix your flavours together to make entirely new creations. If you buy a tobacco flavour that you don't like try mixing it with a different flavour or even another tobacco. Or mix two fruit flavours. There are no rules.

Also try to buy in anticipation of your mood. Maybe you want a dessert flavour for after dinner, a coffee flavour for the evening whilst relaxing or even a fruity flavour for the mornings.

As you vape you will learn how much ml of e-liquid you need to buy. 5-10ml will last a week to two weeks depending on how much you vape. Just make sure you don't run out; you don't want to be tempted to go back to tobacco cigarettes.

What to check for

There are a few things to check before you buy. The PG and VG percentage mix and the nicotine strength are the basics.

A good vendor will also display whether the e-liquid is a known 'tank cracker', contains alcohol and whether the e-liquid contains animal extracts as well as other information.

You should also check that they provide childproof bottles, for obvious reasons.

About tank crackers

Flavours such as cinnamon, citrus fruits and others are known to interact with polycarbonate tanks (polypropylene tanks do not crack). It is the natural acids within the flavours that cause the damage.

Note that it only harms your equipment, NOT YOU!

If you want to have a full choice of e-liquids without worrying about whether it will damage your equipment, buy a Glassomiser or use full stainless steel tanks.

Percentage mixes

You can purchase e-liquid with different percentages of PG and VG. PG is a good flavour carrier and VG produces vapour. A lot of vendors will provide a mix of 70% PG / 30% VG to ensure that the flavour is strong; but it will lack vapour production.

A good balance is 50% PG / 50% VG, which will give you adequate flavour and vapour.

Although it is very tempting to buy e-liquid that has a high VG content in order to get more vapour (e.g. 10% PG / 90% VG) you will find that it is virtually unusable in devices other than rebuildable atomisers.

24 Storing E-liquid

How long does it last?

E-liquid has a shelf life and can remain perfect for up to two years with perfect storage. But realistically you should expect it to expire within 6-12 months.

Manufacturers will (or should) list the expiry date on the bottle, or they might write the date that the e-liquid was created. Proper handling and storage of your e-liquid will help in preventing it from going bad prematurely.

Where to store

Store your e-liquid in a closed box or cupboard and in a place where it is dry and cool. You should not place prefilled cartomisers or e-liquids in an area where it can get warm or where there is light, such as on top of your desk next to your computer or near a window.

E-liquid is greatly affected by light and heat. Flavourings can get hazy and nicotine can degrade when exposed to air, moisture, heat and light. However, PG is not affected by bacteria and viruses as it contains anti-bacterial and anti-fungal substances.

Low temperatures will reduce the oxidation rate and will also help prevent the growth of bacteria and mold. Also, chemical reactions are slowed down so any nicotine will remain fresh for a longer time.

Long term storage

For long term storage it is best to store e-liquid in glass so that it will not be affected by the components of a plastic container. Dark glass bottles are recommended as long term storage containers as the dark colouring of glass bottles helps to prevent light from going through to the e-liquid, keeping it fresh.

The best colour glass to buy is amber.

Plastic bottles are ideal only for short term storage. Plastic bottles may react with the some of the e-liquid ingredients and affect the flavour and quality of your e-liquid.

To refrigerate or not refrigerate

My last point is on storing premixed e-liquid in the refrigerator. I don't personally do it, but some people believe that storing e-liquid this way keeps it fresh; just like food products. But there are two known issues caused by refrigerating or freezing.

The first is that refrigeration may cause condensation, which can lead to bacterial growth and/or a more watery liquid. There will be a small amount of air inside the bottle and it is this air that creates condensation when the bottle is removed from the fridge and left standing at room temperature.

The second is that it will affect the flavourings within most e-liquids; as each flavour will react differently to cold temperatures. So you may find that your e-liquid starts to taste funny or loses its flavour completely.

If you do get into DIY e-liquid then refrigeration or freezing is a different matter for long term storage of pure nicotine, propylene glycol (PG) and vegetable glycerine (VG); as it will prolong their shelf life.

I won't say "don't refrigerate", especially as there are no conclusive tests. But there are **no actual benefits**.

25 Steeping Your E-liquid

Have you bought an e-liquid flavour after you've heard people rave about it? And after you've paid for it, filled your tank and taken a few puffs you think...

..."Ugh, I don't like this, why are people raving about this?"

Maybe your e-liquid needed steeping?

Many people are not aware that most e-liquids need steeping and fail to experience the full potential from their e-liquid because they have not allowed adequate time for it to mature and reach its optimum flavour.

When you buy e-liquid it is unlikely that it has steeped for more than a day or two, as good vendors tend to make their liquids fresh; as opposed to making large quantities that are then put into storage.

Receiving fresh e-liquid is normal, the only problem is that you'll have to wait a little longer to vape it. Many good vendors will actually include instructions as to how long each of their e-liquids will need steeping.

So what is Steeping?

Steeping is the process used to allow the ingredients in your e-liquid to blend and mature, to ensure that you achieve the best possible flavour while you are vaping; steeping also rounds out any harsh flavours.

Steeping your e-liquid is the vaping equivalent of marinating your food or allowing wine to mature.

All flavourings need time to fuse and molecularly bond with the other ingredients such as PG, VG and liquid nicotine.

The more complex the recipe, the more important the steeping process becomes in order to achieve the very best flavour.

While steeping, your e-liquid will normally darken in colour. This shows that the liquid is maturing or has matured. And the higher the nicotine content the darker the e-liquid will become; your e-liquid may also mature more quickly.

Some e-liquids (mainly custards and tobaccos) will never finish steeping. They just keep getting better and better. If you can hold out that long, you'll be able to experience the smoother, deepening flavours for yourself.

Watch out for some fruit flavours, as they can slowly start to lose their flavour over the weeks.

How to Steep

1. Time Steeping

The traditional method of steeping! This is simply done by leaving your bottles in a dark place for one to two days, a week, two weeks or a month. Again, you will need to determine when your e-liquid is ready, by testing it along the way.

The benefit of using this traditional method is that your e-liquid will be naturally steeped. The only disadvantage is that you will need to be patient.

2. Breathing

Breathing is simply removing the cap and dropper and leaving the e-liquid in a cool dark place to mature. It is a faster than steeping, but you may find that your nicotine strength and flavour diminishes slightly.

3. Streathing

This is a combination of 'time steeping' and 'breathing'. You can (on a daily basis) refresh the air in the bottle by removing the cap and squeezing the bottle a few times; allowing the liquid to reach the tip each time.

If you have a glass bottle then just swirl the liquid around in the bottle. After this replace the cap and shake the bottle vigorously, then put it back to mature.

4. Seed Steeping

Not so common is seed steeping. This is where you leave around 10%-20% of the same e-liquid that has already been time steeped for weeks in the bottle; then add fresh e-liquid to the bottle.

This actually speeds up the steeping process of the freshly added e-liquid. And you will see physical (colour) changes within days.

Although you will still need to let the mixture steep, you will not have to wait as long. An e-liquid that may have taken a month to be ready may only take 3-7 days.

How long should I steep my e-liquid?

Sorry... but there is no definitive answer to that question. Only you will be able to answer this through experimentation.

The good news is that once you have experimented with a particular e-liquid once, you will know the exact requirements the next time around.

Some e-liquids are ready to vape straight away (e.g. fruit), some take days and there are some that can take one week (e.g. light tobaccos and creams) to a month or more (e.g. custard and tobaccos flavours) to mature.

Are you in a hurry?

Ok... you've just got your new order of e-liquid. You can't wait to vape them, but they don't taste quite right. The vendor has made them fresh (nothing wrong with that) so they'll need steeping.

But you're not prepared to wait a few days let alone a week. And the thought of waiting a month is totally out of the question.

What do you do?

Well... all hope is not lost. You can opt to do what is known as 'Speed Steeping'. The following methods are the most common (but there are many more).

1. Hot Water Bath

This is the most successful speed steeping method for most people. And you can achieve a 'ready to vape' e-liquid in 4-5 hours as opposed to days or weeks.

Fill a container with hot water up to the base of the neck your e-liquid bottle. Place your bottle into the water and leave until the water cools (luke warm).

You can leave the top on or off; but if you leave the top of make sure the bottle is secure so that it does not tip over.

While the water is cooling you should remove the bottle (two times is adequate) and shake, then put it back.

Once the water has cooled you should repeat the process another two times. The whole process should take around five hours.

2. Ultrasonic cleaner

Now some people swear by these devices. It is relatively easy to do, but can be time consuming depending on which model you have. But once completed you can reduce steeping times by weeks in just a few hours.

If you don't have an ultrasonic (jewellery) cleaner you will have to buy one; which can be costly depending on the model that you choose.

But if your budget is tight you could opt for a mini ultrasonic that they use to clean dentures and small items which will cost less than £10 ($15) online. But you will only be able to fit one or two 10ml bottles in at a time.

The good thing about these machines is that they are also very good at cleaning non electrical equipment. So you can use it to clean your mechanical mods and atomisers.

This method combines two vital functions; vibrations similar to shaking your bottle (from the ultrasonic frequencies) and a warm water bath. It will continuously shake your e-liquid at a level that cannot be achieved manually.

You simply fill the cleaner with water (warm water if it does not have a heating feature) and then place your bottle (or bottles) into the cleaner.

Now the time consuming factor is that these machines have timers that you will need to keep resetting. So if your machine has a 3 minute timer and you are going to steep your e-liquid for 5 hours you will need to reset the machine 100 times... Yep! You read that right.

3. Microwave

This is the easiest of the methods, but I have found that that it changes the flavour dramatically. Microwaves do not always heat food evenly and I have found this to be the same when heating e-liquids.

It is also advisable to use glass bottles not plastic bottles; as it is not clear how the plastic and e-liquid ingredients react together in a microwave.

Simply pop your bottle into the microwave. Heat the liquid for no more than 8 seconds. Remove, shake for as long as you can and leave it to cool. Some people repeat this 2-3 tomes. But as I stated earlier I have found that it changes the flavour.

It's your choice as to which method you decide to choose. But I have found that nothing beats 'good ole' time steeping.

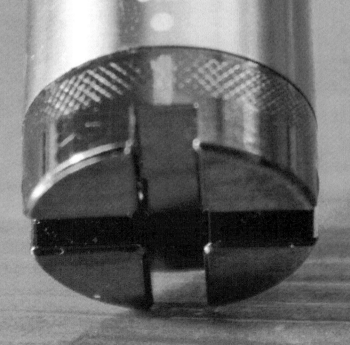

AND FINALLY...

26 Don't get ripped off

I unfortunately hear so many stories about people being charged extortionate prices for equipment and e-liquid. Electronic cigarettes, personal vaporisers and e-liquid have become a big market, soon to be damaged by excessive regulations.

But with all growing industries you'll get unscrupulous individuals looking to take advantage and make a quick buck. If you're about to buy your first kit or you've been burnt by the buying process, my main advice to you is this...

... Do your research!

By now you should have an idea of what you're looking for in terms of equipment.

I started off with a 900mah 'eGo style' battery, a CE4 clearomiser and a USB charger. It cost me £6.99 ($11) from Ebay.

I then bought three more clearomisers for £3.70 ($6) (also from Ebay) and I was set. It allowed me to get use to vaping and quit tobacco cigarettes for good.

How much!?!

Imagine if I added another battery, a case and a wall charger to my set up. Realistically that should cost me less than £12 ($19).

But I know people who have been stung for between £100 ($155) and £150 ($233) for a basic set up commonly consisting of two eGo batteries, two clearomisers, a USB and wall charger, a case and two bottles of e-liquid. Shocking!

For those prices the equipment would need to be gold plated and you would be serving me the finest whisky.

These problems mostly happen in vaping shops, but I don't want you to think that all vape shops are bad; because they're not. They need to make a profit just like any other business and they have overheads to cover.

Don't buy on impulse!

Go to a shop, see what they have to offer, then go home and research it. If you're happy with their price go back. A good vape shop will talk you through using the equipment and make sure you're happy and most importantly safe.

Watch and see how they deal with customers. If it's all sales talk and no real advice, walk away.

The internet is your friend, especially Ebay, YouTube and Google. Yes Ebay has clones and no name brands but you pay clone or no name brand prices and they work just as well (some vape shops also sell clones so keep that in mind). These sites will help you to establish the right price you should be paying for the equipment you want to buy, learn more about the equipment before you buy it and also help you to research companies.

Take baby steps

Just like when you first start to drive and you buy a 'run around'... buy some clones. Once you've done your experimenting with equipment go and buy the originals (if you want) from reputable companies.

Don't get caught up in the clone v original debate; buy what suits your pockets. The most important thing should be that you stay off tobacco cigarettes.

If I were to do it over again knowing what I know now I would still start off with my first setup. £10.69 ($17) is a small investment for finding out whether I liked vaping. I would then move onto a variable voltage/wattage device like a Vamo with the CE4 clearomisers and then onto RBAs and mechanical mods.

When it comes to e-liquid unless it's a gourmet brand most companies are offering the same thing. I'm afraid its trial and error here. This is why I started making my own e-liquid. Taste is subjective so (if you can) try before you buy or buy small sample sizes.

27 Quitting Nicotine Completely

If you want to reduce or eliminate your dependency on nicotine, electronic cigarettes are a great way to achieve this. In fact you'll find it an easy and painless process.

And if you're like me, quitting 'cold turkey' was not an option.

Now the great thing is that you are in total control of how and when you want to achieve your goals. Whether you want to continue vaping because you enjoy the flavours and the action of vaping or you want to be 'smoking and vaping' free... the choice is yours!

However, for this to work, you'll need to give up tobacco cigarettes... completely!

With any of these methods you will need to construct a plan. Set a start and end date that you feel you can stick to. If you've smoked for a very long time you'll need to create a plan with a longer time span.

Method 1:

This is where you reduce the nicotine strength of your e-liquid over a period of time. You stay on a planned nicotine level for a set period of time and then reduce the level and stay on that for a set period of time.

You decide how long you want stay on each level and how long you want to take to reach your desired nicotine level.

If you find that the date is approaching for you to go down to the next level (let's say 12mg) but you still have e-liquid left (e.g. 18mg), use it; even if you have to adjust your plan slightly. Otherwise you'll just end up using it later, when you should be on a lower level.

Or you could give it away (smiley face)!

You may want to consider reducing your levels based on finishing a bottle of e-liquid 'around' a certain date as opposed to cutting suddenly on a specific date.

Your plan might look something like this:

- June 1st – 14th: 24mg
- June 15th – 30th: 18mg
- July 1st – 31st: 12mg
- August 1st – 14th: 6mg
- August 15th – 31st: 3mg
- September 1st: 0 mg

Method 2:

This method is where you use two different strength e-liquids at the same time. This allows you to still get a 'kick' at certain times of the day while getting your body use to a lower intake of nicotine. I know that in the mornings I needed to 'get my fix'.

Ok! That sounds wrong, but you know what I mean...

... Moving on!

So you may have one e-liquid at 18mg and another at 12mg. You might decide to use the stronger strength only in the mornings and use the lower strength for the rest of the day. Or choose to use the higher strength only after meals. Go for what you know you be able to commit to.

You can reduce these strengths down to zero or a relatively low level as time goes by in your plan; so 12mg and 6mg, 8mg and 3mg etc.

Your plan might look something like this:

- June 1st – 14th: 24mg / 18mg
- June 15th – 30th: 18mg / 12mg
- July 1st – 31st: 12mg / 6mg
- August 1st – 14th: 6mg / 3mg
- August 15th – 31st: 3mg / 0mg
- September 1st: 0 mg

Which one should you use?

The choice is yours as to which method you opt to use. You might even come up with your own.

Start with the nicotine strength that you are comfortable with, it doesn't have to be 24mg. Don't be afraid to adjust or extend your plan as time goes by if you notice that you're having problems sticking with it; you can even mix the methods.

I spent a longer time than planned at 12mg before moving down to 8mg (this is where I used method 2 for a while).

Move at your own pace!

The important thing to remember is that you've freed yourself from tobacco cigarettes and the 4000+ harmful chemicals they contain.

28 Vaping Dehydration

Have you ever watched a vaping video and seen the presenter pause to gulp back pure water? The very first time I saw this I thought... "Oh! Can't he wait until after?"

Back then I wasn't aware that vaping can cause dehydration, but my ignorance slowly diminished when I noticed that I was drinking a lot more water than before and went in search of answers. Dehydration is common amongst vapers and it doesn't take long to develop.

But why?

Of the few ingredients in e-liquids we can confidently point the finger at Propylene Glycol. PG molecules love water and attract and hold onto (or bond with) water molecules. So while you vape, the PG in your e-liquid is removing water from your saliva, mouth, throat, nose and other parts in that general area.

If you stay hydrated whilst vaping this is not a problem, but if you continuously ignore your body's need to increase water intake and reduce water loss it can lead to serious health issues.

In the early stages of dehydration there are three common signs amongst vapers; thirst, a dry mouth and dark coloured urine. Other symptoms may include tiredness, headaches, dizziness and loss of strength, lack of stamina and dry lips or eyes.

At this stage dehydration can easily be reversed by drinking more water. However, ignoring all of these signs (over a long period of time) and not increasing your water intake can lead to kidney problems, kidney stones, constipation, cholesterol and liver problems; as well as muscle and joint damage.

Let's go back to 'dry mouth' for a moment.

From experience, having a dry mouth changes the way your e-liquid tastes. After spending so much time finding flavours, I want to enjoy what I'm vaping. So I always have plain water to hand.

You should avoid fizzy, flavoured or sugary drinks as well as coffee, tea and alcohol; as these can actually contribute to dehydration.

The other issues with a dry mouth are tooth decay and halitosis. Dryness in the mouth stimulates bacterial growth leading to tooth decay and bad breath (which is also a problem for tobacco smokers as well).

Stay hydrated by drinking plain water throughout the day.

29 Understanding Vapers Tongue

So you've loaded up your favourite e-liquid, started vaping and... wait a minute! You can't taste anything. You try again.

Still no flavour!

You change your e-liquid, your clearomiser, or your wick in your rebuildable atomiser... nothing! You even change your coil... still nothing! What's happening?

Well don't worry... it sounds like you have 'Vapers Tongue'.

Vapers tongue is the more popular name used by the vaping community for a temporary non-fatal condition called 'olfactory fatigue'.

Your tongue is not broken and you'll be able to taste food and drinks normally. It's just your vaping that's affected. It will go away naturally in a few days or weeks; just like a cold. But can you wait several days or weeks?

It's not the nicest experience; not being able to taste your favourite flavoured e-liquid and it can be worrying the first time that it happens to you.

What happened to the flavour?

We all assume that we taste with our tongue. In actual fact your tongue receptors can only taste five things: sweet, sour, salty, bitter, and umami (savoury).

Your tongue does not actually taste the complex flavours within your food or drinks. But it works in conjunction with your olfactory receptors at the top of your nasal passage, to produce the final flavour.

This close relationship between your tongue receptors and your olfactory receptors is most noticeable when you have a head cold.

Your food tastes different when your sense of smell is impaired.

What is really being affected is the flavour of your food (the combination of taste and smell). You are only detecting the taste and not the food odours.

Taste itself is focused on distinguishing chemicals that have a sweet, salty, sour, bitter, or umami taste. Interaction between the sense of taste and smell enhance our perception of the food we eat.

You taste some of the vapour with your tongue, but your sense of smell is what allows you to experience the flavour of your e-liquid.

What causes 'Vapers Tongue'?

There can be any number of reasons why you might get 'Vapers Tongue'. I had my first experience two months after I started vaping. Thankfully I knew what it was, but I had to do some research to learn how to deal with it.

1. Not Switching Flavours

If you're vaping the same flavour for days, weeks or even months on end without switching it up, your olfactory receptors can become temporarily desensitised.

Just like a fish market worker becomes desensitised to the strong smell of the fish; with constant exposure, the strong smell eventually disappears.

2. Quitting Smoking

If you are a new vaper, you WILL get 'Vapers Tongue' but it may only last a few hours or days (as opposed to weeks and months). This is because smoking dulls your sense of taste and smell.

When you first start vaping you may wonder what all the fuss is about in regards to certain flavours that people have raved about and you've tried. After several weeks your senses start to improve because you are no longer smoking and you start to taste the full flavour of your e-liquid.

During this transition and as your senses start to return, your olfactory system may overload, causing it to become confused or it may completely shut down, causing 'Vapers Tongue'. This can happen several times during your transition from smoking.

3. Colds or Allergies

Problems with your sinuses and your nasal passages will affect your sense of smell. Your olfactory receptors cannot do their job. There is nothing you can do about this other than get rid of your cold or take medication for your allergies.

If you've always had problems with taste due to sinus issues then you could opt to vape unflavoured e-liquid.

4. Dehydration

Vaping dehydrates your body, especially your mouth area. If too much moisture is removed it results in a dry mouth and a thin film can form on your tongue and nasal passages, which can affect your sense of taste.

5. None of the above

As I stated before, there could be any a number of reasons why you might get 'Vapers Tongue'. However, the four listed above are the most common.

Getting rid of 'Vapers Tongue'

There are some wild and crazy methods being suggested on the Internet, so careful about the methods you try in order to rid yourself of vapers tongue.

Putting cotton wool in your mouth WILL NOT cure 'Vapers Tongue', neither will going back to tobacco cigarettes out of frustration. Yes! I've heard it all... hopefully!

Here are some **sensible** methods which are known to work.

1. Reset your receptors

This method has been used for hundreds of years by perfumers, tea buyers and spice merchants to name a few. They will shock their olfactory receptors into "resetting".

All you need to do is open a bag of freshly ground coffee and take several deep inhales. Do not to inhale the actual coffee grinds. The unique molecular structure of the coffee odorants does the "resetting".

2. Rotate you flavours

Try not to waste anymore of your favourite e-liquid. Try some strong flavours like mint or menthol to shock your senses.

Also this is the perfect time to use up those flavours that you don't like. The ones that you still see in your cupboard and cause you to groan and think of the money you wasted. You can't taste them now but they still contain nicotine.

Find a few new favourites (maybe not while you have 'Vapers Tongue') it will help to keep it away in the future.

Ensure that the flavours you vape are drastically different. For example don't have all coffee or all tobacco e-liquids. Mix it up! Fruit, dessert, mints, menthol, drinks, tobacco, creams... you get the gist.

3. Drink a lot of water

Water is good for you, so not only will you be eliminating possible dehydration but also looking after your body and preventing a film build up in your nasal passage.

4. Take care of your mouth

Brush your teeth and tongue, gargle with a minty mouthwash and chew minty gum to help cleanse your pallet, and keep your mouth moist throughout the day.

5. Other methods

Other methods include vaping unflavoured e-liquid, gargling vinegar, drinking lemon water, sucking a lemon and chewing ginger.

30 Conclusion

So there you have it! You now have enough information to confidently buy and maintain your first (or even second) set of equipment. And you'll be prepared for the most common issues that come with vaping. Whether they are equipment, e-liquid or health related.

Take your time and don't overdo it... vaping all day is not advised. Vaping is fun but don't forget that it still contains nicotine. So take a few minutes to vape (or a few puffs) then **put it down...**easier said than done.

Enjoy your vaping journey!

Thank You!

...for choosing this book!

If you enjoyed it or found it useful,
would you be kind enough to
leave a review on Amazon?

It would be greatly appreciated!

Acknowledgements

First and foremost I want to acknowledge the continuous support and encouragement from my family. Especially you Verona!
You are truly a Godsend!

I would also like to acknowledge and thank everyone else who contributed to this book.

Special thanks to:

Sophie Carrera Photography
for their initial photography of my equipment

The following three images were provided under the Creative Commons 2.0 licence
https://creativecommons.org/licenses/by/2.0/legalcode

Page -1
'Smoking' by Nicoletta Ciunci
https://www.flickr.com/photos/svaboda/5286271830

Page 80
'Eliquid containers at a vape shop' by Lindsay Fox
https://www.flickr.com/photos/87735223@N02/9631728028

Page 120
'Smoke-Fall' by Sodanie Chea
https://www.flickr.com/photos/sodaniechea/8819220638

www.evguides.co.uk

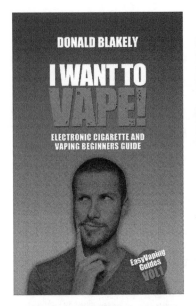

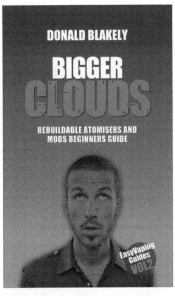

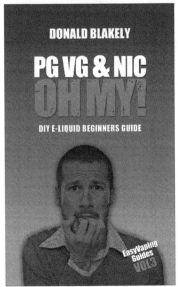

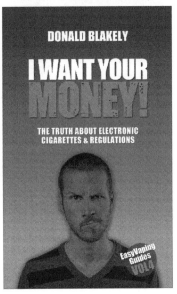

Made in the USA
Middletown, DE
13 June 2022